Gluten Intolerance -
more than just a diet trend!
Symptoms may mimic other diseases,
thus the term

The Masquerader
CELIAC DISEASE

By Barbara Neal Jones
Forward by Subhash Gumber, MD, PHD

ACKNOWLEDGMENTS

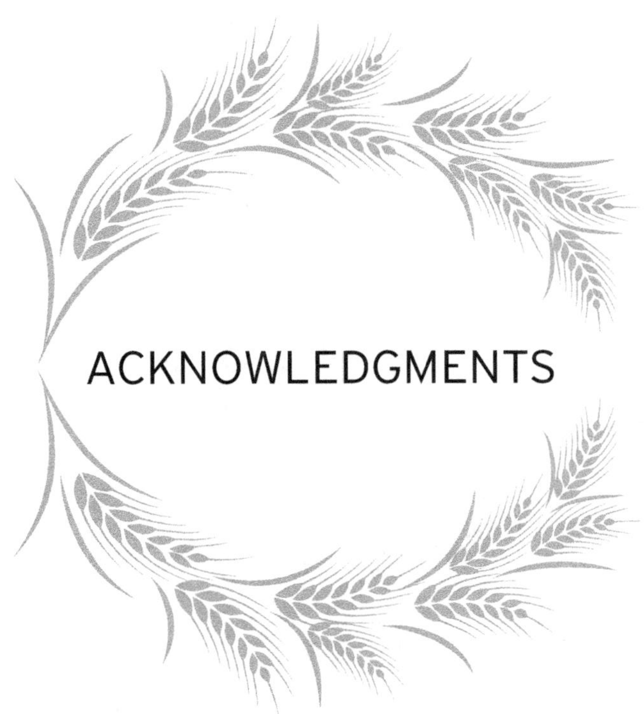

My very special thanks to Dr. Gumber's nurse practitioner, Audrey Avitable, who offered invaluable suggestions for the book.

Also to my daughter Toni Kaplan, who is a registered nurse, and after reading the first draft offered her most appreciated professional opinion.

I am also very grateful to my son-in-law, Donnie James who, after reading the final draft, gave me some very sound advise. His opinion from the perspective of the average person, inspired me to make some changes. These changes would allow the message of the book to be better understood by the layman. The person who has helped me in every way possible, is my daughter, Dana James. Dana is my business manager, as well as the artist who drew the illustrations in the book. Dana has always given much needed support for the book and all the medical problems caused by Celiac Desease. I thank her so much for that.

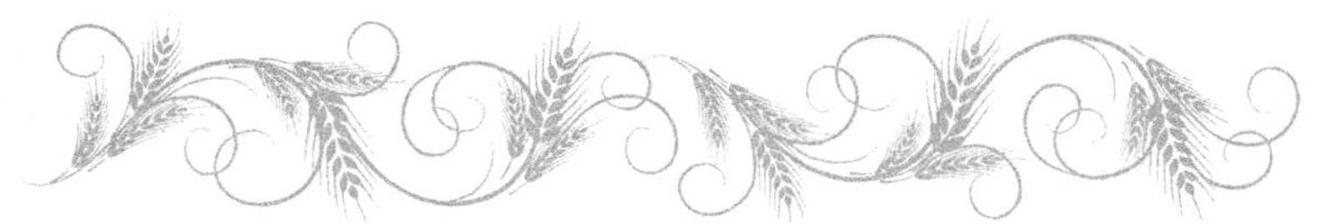

CONTENTS

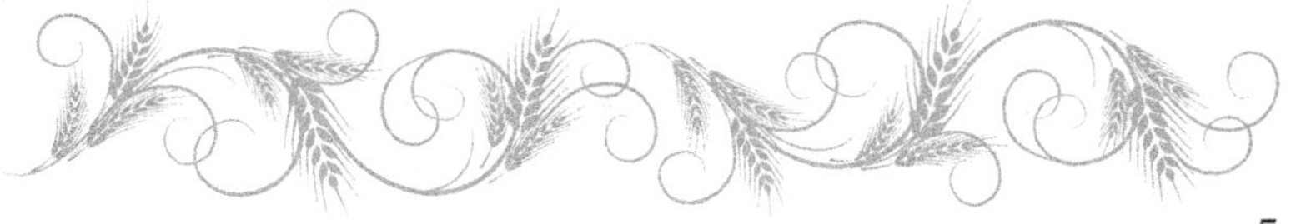

FORWARD

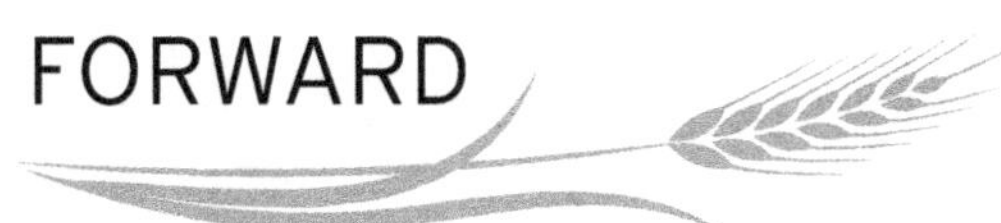

Celiac disease is an under-diagnosed condition with some estimates suggesting that as many as 1 in 250 people have a gluten allergy or intolerance. Many people have suffered for years before an accurate diagnosis is made. All too frequently, other diagnoses are made before arriving at the right one. I have personally seen patients' lives change for the better once the accurate diagnosis is made. Diagnosis is made with blood tests and confirming small intestinal biopsies. The diagnosis is then confirmed when gluten is eliminated from the diet and symptoms resolve. People's lives change in unimaginable ways. Barbara Jones' life changed before my eyes: She became a different person. She wrote this book to help others, who like her, have celiac disease and want to live a better life.

Subhash Gumber, M.D., PhD.
Managing Partner, Raleigh/Cary Medical Group
Gastroenterology and Wake Endoscopy Center

INTRODUCTION

Celiac disease ("celiac") is an autoimmune digestive disease, characterized by a permanent intolerance to gluten. Celiac is considered an autoimmune disorder because the body's immune system malfunctions and attacks the body's own tissues and organs. When a person with celiac ingests gluten (i.e., the protein contained in wheat, rye, oats and barley), their immune system triggers an inflammatory reaction in the lining of the small intestine. The cells that normally line the walls of the small intestine are elongated villi (finger-like projections) that allow absorption of nutrients. When food containing gluten is ingested, the surface of the small intestine is damaged, and the elongated shape of the villi becomes flattened, resulting in less surface area for nutrient absorption (see figures A&B/images 1&2 on the next page). Nutrients are then passed through the small intestine rather than absorbed. As a result, there are a number of diverse and supposedly unrelated symptoms that can cause ill health for a short time if diagnosed early, or for a lifetime if not properly diagnosed.

The following drawings of hands with arrows following the fingers allow you to visualize the surface area for absorption of nutrients.

Figure A – The outstretched fingers show how much more area for absorption is found in the normal small intestine.

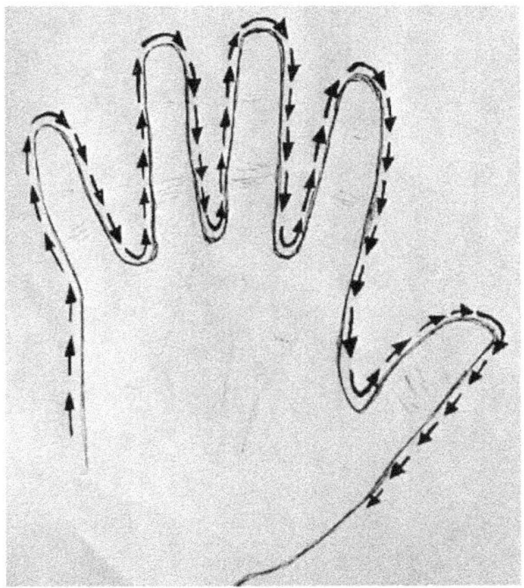

Figure B – The closed fist demonstrates how gluten affects the small intestine lining.

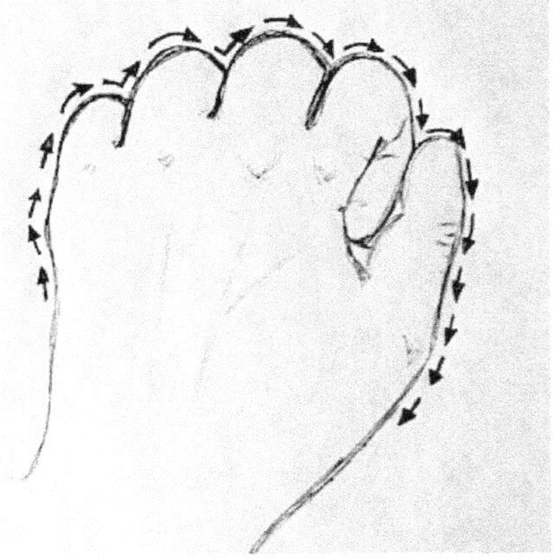

The following images demonstrate biopsies of cells found in the small intestine. Note the "flattened" area of the cells in Image 2 – a small intestine that has been effected by celiac.

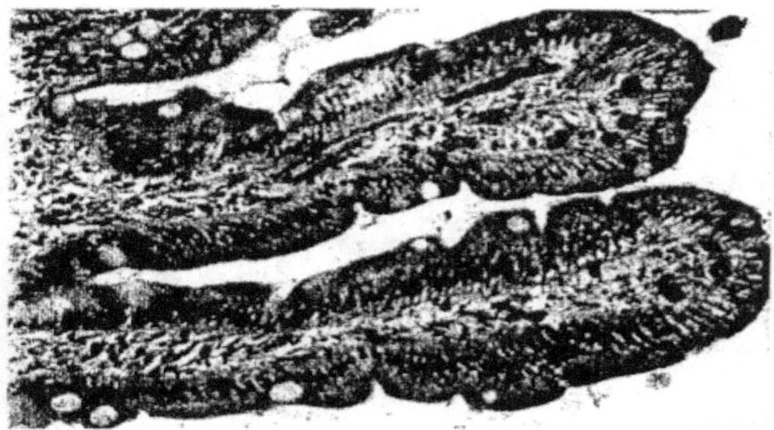

Image 1 – Normal small intestine villi. The elongated shape of the villi increases the surface area for absorption.

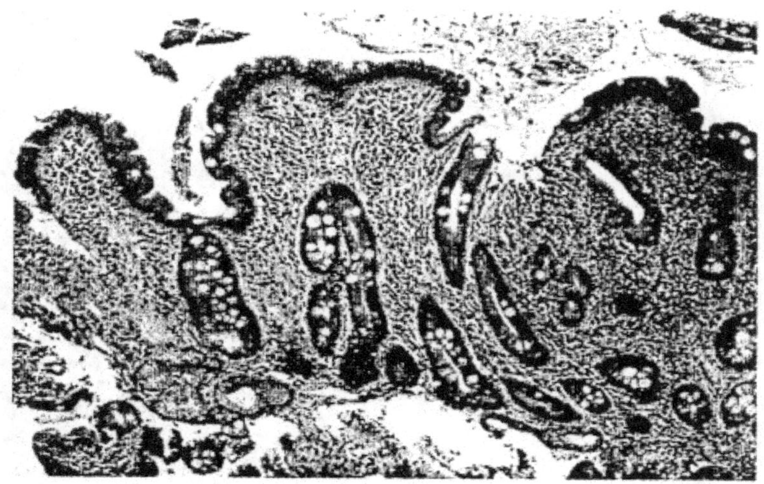

Image 2 – Atrophied small intestine villi due to gluten intolerance. The flattened, wide villi result in reduced surface area for absorption.

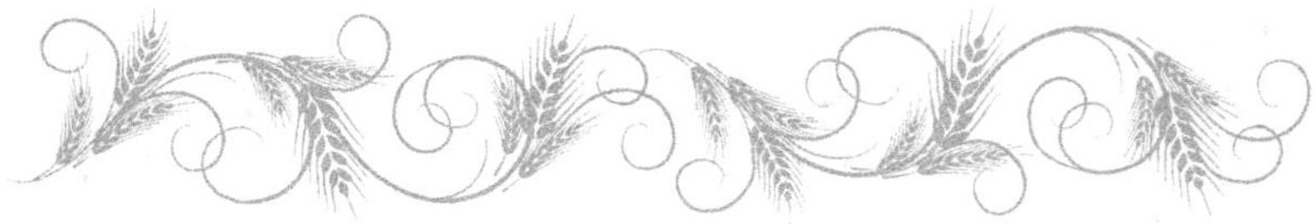

The Masquerader

Millions of people log onto the internet seeking information about health issues. Unfortunately, everyone in this country and around the world does not have access to a computer. Even if they do, the task of putting together the diverse symptoms they are experiencing may be too daunting for some people.

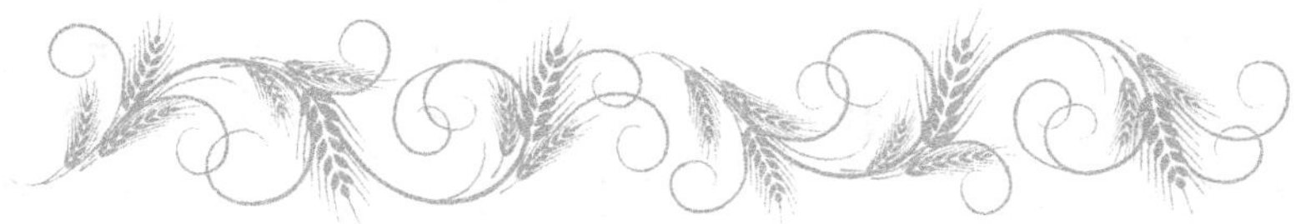

The symptoms that are causing you a problem may seem too insignificant to put together to form the picture of celiac, an autoimmune disease. I refer to it in this book as "the Masquerader" because it masquerades as so many different illnesses, which can potentially lead to a misdiagnosis. For me, the symptoms included gas, recurring abdominal pain and bloating, and chronic malodorous diarrhea, which led to a diagnosis of Irritable Bowel Syndrome ("IBS"). I also suffered from anemia with accompanying fatigue, tingling and numbness in my legs, bone and joint pain, muscle cramps, and later, seizures. All of this seemed unrelated, and it wasn't until years later, when I was diagnosed with celiac, that it all came together for me.

You should not diagnose yourself, but when armed with information that can help you know what questions to ask your doctor about the symptoms you are having, you can potentially regain good health. Hopefully my experience will help you realize that these different sets of symptoms are important and should be discussed with your doctor. This book is meant to be a guide to help with your quest for good health. There is a lot of information that can be used to aid in a diagnosis, and if the diagnosis is celiac, the treatment can be as easy as a change in diet. I do not mean to simplify the diet. It is very stringent and causes major changes in life style; but with time, it becomes second nature. However, if a person with celiac does not know they have the condition they can suffer – really suffer – for years. Even people with access to the internet will benefit from the concise way the information is presented and can share it with people who would otherwise have never heard of celiac.

The idea for this book came to me a year or so after I was diagnosed with celiac disease. At the time I did not use the internet and there were no books on the shelves of main stream book stores pertaining to celiac. There were a number of books about diabetes, crohn's disease, lupus, etc. But to learn about celiac, it was necessary to go to the health food store or specialty store. For me, that would probably not happen. There was no reason for me to search for a disease I had never heard of because at that time most doctors in the U.S. were not looking for it either. In some countries, where celiac is recognized early, the diagnosis is usually made within 2 to 3 weeks after onset of symptoms. For example, in a country like Italy, this vigilance results in early diagnosis. In the United States, the time between the first symptoms and diagnosis averages about 10 years.

Recognizing celiac can be difficult because some of the symptoms are similar to those of other diseases. Sometimes celiac disease is confused with IBS, iron deficiency, anemia, crohn's disease, diverticulitis, intestinal infections and chronic fatigue syndrome. There can be serious neurological problems caused by celiac that health care professionals may not realize are related to the disease. Celia disease is commonly misdiagnosed in the U.S., thus the term "the Masquerader."

SYMPTOMS

SYMPTOMS

Symptoms of celiac disease may include one or more of the following:

- Gas
- Recurring abdominal bloating and pain
- Chronic diarrhea
- Constipation
- Pale, foul-smelling, fatty stool
- Weight loss/weight gain
- Fatigue
- Unexplained anemia (a low count of red blood cells causing fatigue)
- Bone or joint pain
- Osteoporosis
- Osteopenia
- Behavioral changes
- Tingling numbness in legs (from nerve damage)
- Muscle cramps
- Seizures
- Missed menstrual periods (often because of excessive weight loss)
- Infertility
- Recurrent miscarriages
- Delayed growth
- Failure to thrive in infants
- Pale sores inside the mouth called apthous ulcers
- Tooth discoloration or loss of enamel
- Itchy skin rash called dermatitis herpetiformis

A person with celiac disease may have no symptoms. People without symptoms are still at risk for complications from the disease, including malnutrition. The longer one goes undiagnosed and untreated, the greater the chance of developing malnutrition and other complications. Anemia, delayed growth and weight loss are signs of malnutrition – the body is just not getting enough nutrients. Malnutrition is a serious problem for children because they need adequate nutrition to develop properly; this could result in short stature.

ASSOCIATED AUTO-IMMUNE DISEASES

- Addison's Disease
- Insulin Dependent Diabetes (Type I)
- Pernicious Anemia (Deficiency of Vitamin B12)
- Raynaud's Phenomenon
- Scleroderma
- Sjogen's Syndrome
- Systematic Lupus Erythematosus
- Thyroid Disease
    - 1-Grave's Disease (overactive thyroid gland)
    - 2-Hashimoto's Disease (underactive thyroid gland)

INDIVIDUALS AT INCREASED RISK

INDIVIDUALS AT INCREASED RISK

Individuals at increased risk of celiac disease are those with:
- Type 1 diabetes mellitus
- Thyroid disease
- Down syndrome
- Chronic Diarrhea
- Unexplained short stature
- Infertility
- Anemia
- Lactose intolerance
- Family history of celiac disease or dermatitis herpeti-formis "Dermatitis Herpetiformis" is an associated skin condition characterized by a blistering rash and sever itching. There is usually intestinal damage even if digestive symptoms are absent. Drug treatment may be helpful to relieve itching; however, the celiac diet must be strictly followed as that is the only way to treat celiac disease.

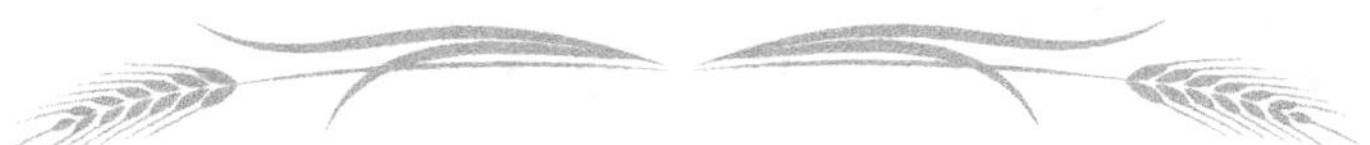

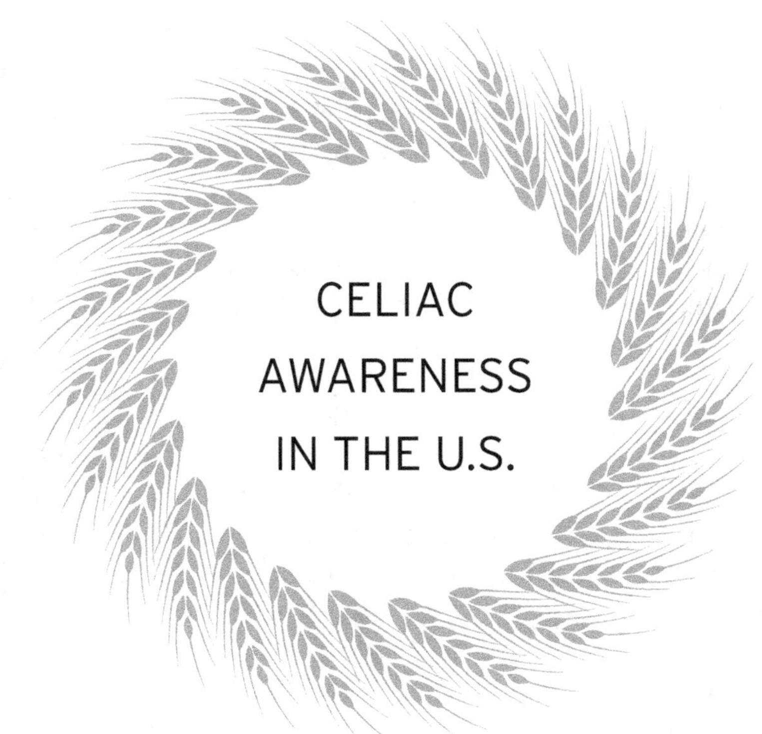

CELIAC AWARENESS IN THE U.S.

Sometimes celiac disease is triggered, or becomes active for the first time, after a traumatic event such as surgery, pregnancy, child birth, viral infections or severe emotional stress.

I am sure that my trigger in my fifties was severe upper back pain that became almost unbearable. My primary care doctor thought it was musculo- skeletal pain and referred me to a physical therapist. One very smart physical therapist suggested I see a cardiologist. I am sure she saved my life. The pain was angina. Within a few days, I had double bypass open heart surgery. I was on the brink of a major heart attack. The same week that I had heart surgery, I received a diagnosis of celiac disease. I am so grateful for both of the diagnoses and both treatments. One saved my life, the other, with a drastic change in diet, made life much more pleasant.

A diagnosis of celiac does not cost money for new medications; it only requires determination to eat what is healthy for you. The good news is that a lifetime gluten-free diet can completely stop the autoimmune response. The classic case of celiac disease that was taught in medical school was that of a child with diarrhea, abdominal bloating and pain. However, many people do not develop symptoms of the disease until adulthood. Now it is recognized as a lifelong condition that can be diagnosed at any age, even in the elderly.

Celiac disease can affect anyone. However, it is a genetically inherited disease and tends to occur in families of European descent. Celiac is one of the most common diseases in Europe, with a prevalence of 1 in every 250 to 300 people, according to "Communique", a Mayo Reference Services Publication.

Over thirty years ago, I read a book by Adelle Davis, "Let's Eat Right To Keep Fit." That book became my Bible for Nutrition. It is old and tattered – held together with a rubber band. Reading it for the first time in my early thirties, I thought a lot of her examples must be greatly exaggerated. Even though she was a highly respected author and expert on nutrition, I could not imagine people having such extreme reactions to an inadequate diet. I was to find out first-hand how accurate she was.

There are hundreds of books that explain the value of good nutrition. I referred to some of them to be sure I was giving my family the best food to promote good health. Today, the books about supplements interest me the most, because reading down the lists of vitamins and minerals and seeing how their lack can affect your health is astounding to me. When I was diagnosed with celiac disease, it made so much sense. I had been eating healthy foods, but with a malabsorption problem the nutrients were passing through and I was getting very little benefit from them.

Some people are diagnosed in a matter of months, some in a number of years. As noted earlier, the median time for diagnosis of celiac is ten years. My case is obviously different, as it took around forty years for me to be diagnosed. Now, with more awareness and reference materials, people can find help much quicker. With celiac disease becoming more widely known, many of you may not have to experience so many of the symptoms that I did. After being diagnosed with celiac, the most frightening consequence of eating anything containing gluten was the possibility of developing cancer. This word would deter even those of us with the least amount of will power. Some people have died of the disease due to the development of intestinal lymphoma, but these are mainly adults who have severe celiac disease at the outset. Something else that keeps me on a strict diet is the possibility of fecal incontinence (i.e., uncontrollable diarrhea). This is a real possibility for those of us who struggle with adhering to the diet over an extended period of time. But today, due to an on-going trend for people to avoid having wheat in their diets as a dietary choice, there are so many gluten-free products and restaurants catering to this trend with gluten-free menus, that the diet can be fairly easily managed.

There is an important distinction between making a dietary choice to eliminate wheat versus having a wheat-gluten intolerance – celiac disease is an intolerance to gluten and can be life threatening. It's a medical condition that requires an altered diet, with no exposure to gluten. Unfortunately, most people aren't aware that gluten is found in everyday items like soy sauce, beer, crackers, cereal, and even non-food items like glue on envelopes. For more examples see the section titled "helpful tips and information."

THE TIMELINE FOR THE PROGRESSION OF MY DISEASE

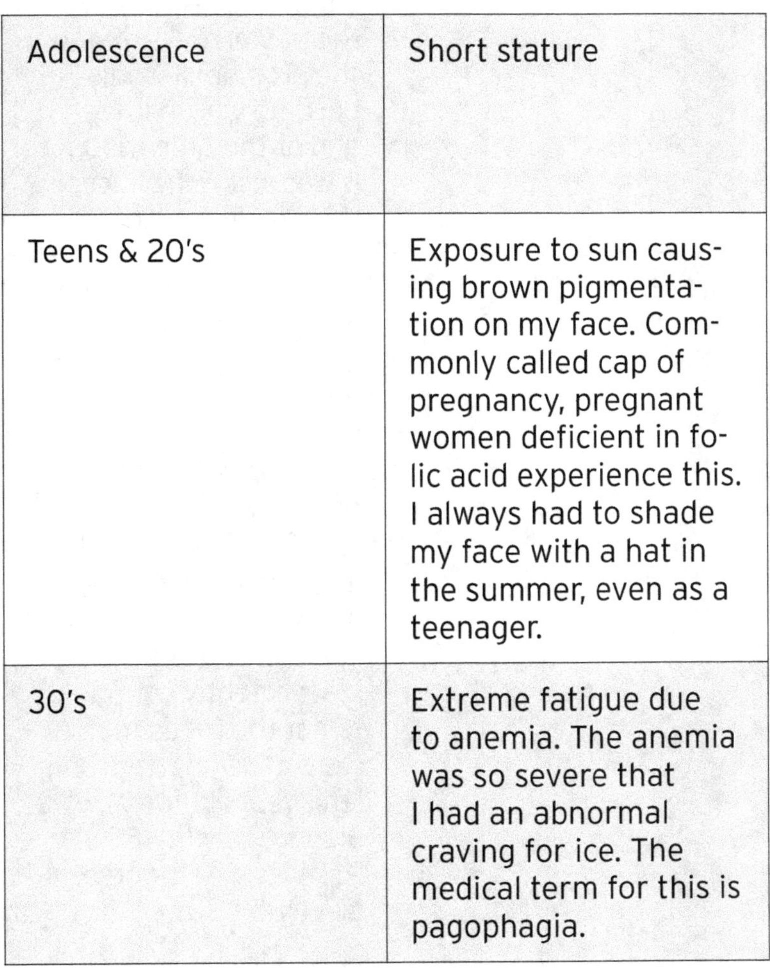

Adolescence	Short stature
Teens & 20's	Exposure to sun causing brown pigmentation on my face. Commonly called cap of pregnancy, pregnant women deficient in folic acid experience this. I always had to shade my face with a hat in the summer, even as a teenager.
30's	Extreme fatigue due to anemia. The anemia was so severe that I had an abnormal craving for ice. The medical term for this is pagophagia.

40's	**Abdominal bloating** – after a normal meal I looked like I was a few months pregnant. **Nausea** – going out to eat Italian, especially the pasta, exacerbated the problem. I would become very nauseated and at the time thought it was just rich sauces that made me sick.
Early 50's	Diarrhea was the bane of my existence as it became more and more frequent. But more than the frequency, I also learned that malodorous stools where a significant sign of celiac. It was very frustrating and very embarrassing. Until I was diagnosed, I inadvertently continued to eat the foods that were causing the problem. Years before, I was diagnosed with IBS, but this was much worse than IBS. I have also experienced some bone pain that is one of the symptoms of celiac disease.

Late 50's	Gastroesophageal reflux ("GERD") caused me enough concern that I saw a specialist. Dr. Gumber, my gastroenterologist, did an endoscopy and it was during this test that I was diagnosed with celiac disease as well as GERD. During the endoscopy procedure, a tube was inserted through the mouth and esophagus to view the esophagus, stomach, and small intestine. Doctor Gumber noted that the lining of the small intestine was abnormal and took biopsies from that site. There are blood tests that can be performed, but a biopsy of the small intestine is needed for confirmation. BIOPSY OF THE SMALL INSTESTINE IS THE GOLD STANDARD FOR DIAGNOSIS OF CELIAC DISEASE.

60's	During the past several years I have experienced mild seizures that are controlled by medication. It is known that gluten sensitivity can cause seizure disorders. Screening for celiac disease should be considered in patients with unexplained neurological disorders such as seizures, ataxia, dementia, etc.

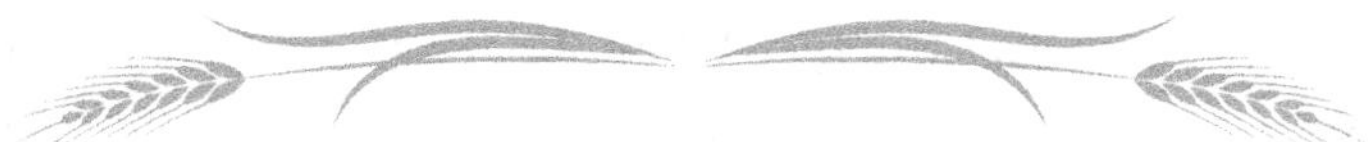

HELPFUL TIPS AND INFORMATION

1. It is extremely important to continue with your normal eating habits before being tested for celiac. If gluten has been eliminated from your diet before testing, the results may be inaccurate.

2. Extra vitamins may be taken. However, gluten restricted diets may continue to be inadequate in B vitamins.

3. Gluten can also be found in non-food products. Examples are lipstick, medicine, vitamins, stamps and glue on envelopes.

4. One word that crops up quite often is malt. It is found in most cereals and some candy. You will see gluten free on the boxes of a few cereals that are allowed. Be careful with candy though. Any candy that is a crunch or crispy is a no-no.

5. When using your own recipes for cookies, cakes, etc., with gluten-free flour, be sure to use xanthum gum to get the right consistency. It is a little pricey, but very necessary. Make sure to check the label on the flour, it could contain xanthum gum, if not you will have to add it.

6. People with celiac disease have to be extremely careful about what they buy for lunch at school or work, what they purchase at the grocery store, what they eat at restaurants or parties, or what they grab for a snack. When invited for dinner at someone's house, be sure to let them know about your gluten allergy so there will be food prepared that you can eat.

7. Usually the better the restaurant, the more control the chef has over the ingredients. When in doubt, it is always best to ask the server. Let them know why you are asking and they will make it a point to find out for sure if there is gluten in the food you've ordered. There is always the possibility for cross contamination when gluten-free foods are prepared in the same kitchen as foods containing gluten. Ask if the restaurant has an area devoted solely to gluten-free food prep.

8. Gluten can be found in foods as a basic ingredient or as a result of preparation or processing. Reading labels is extremely important. Foods with unknown composition should not be included in the diet (e.g., like a hotdog).

9. There are a number of gluten free foods that are delicious, such as rice pasta, gluten free crackers, cookies, waffles and many more. There are entire sections in most grocery stores devoted to gluten free foods.

10. A word of encouragement. With practice, screening for gluten becomes second nature. You will find that eating becomes as natural as it was before the diagnosis of celiac.

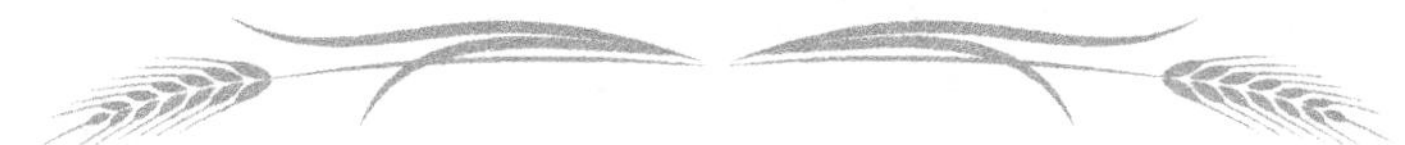

FABULOUS GLUTEN-FREE RECIPES

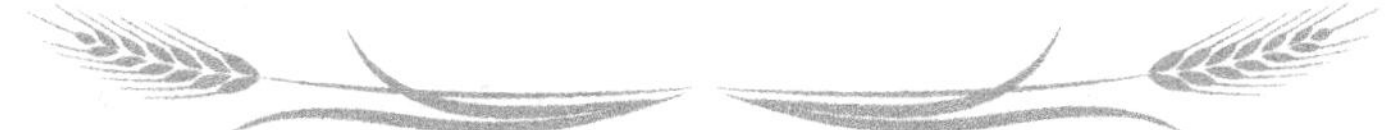

I am sure you will enjoy these recipes – they are presented in such an interesting way. The commentary from our fellow celiac in Australia, Allan Gardyne, gives a flare to what would otherwise be ordinary recipes. With his kind permission I have included them here.

By: Allan Gardyne - with a lot of help from his wife, Joanna, who looked after the weekly lifestyle/recipes section of the Fraser Coast Chronicle for several years. *"My recipes include scrumptious, easy-to-make, meals, a cake or three, plenty of delicious snacks, puddings, an unusual soup, and even a fudge recipe. My favorite recipe is a fabulous gluten-free fruit-cake, concocted by Joanna after many dedicated hours of experimenting. I have a sweet tooth, so I've included a few chewy, sweet treats."*

1. Joanna's Chicken Casserole
2. Cheese Sauce (with butter)
3. Savoury Rice Bake
4. Salmon and Rice Soufflé
5. Cheesy Potato and Ham Casserole
6. Pork with Cherry Almond Sauce
7. Asparagus in Crab Sauce
8. Fast Beef Stroganoff
9. Bacon, Potato and Onion Pie
10. Salmon and Potato Bake
11. Tropical Chicken
12. Rice Tomato Pilaf
13. Easy Salmon Frittata
14. Rich, Moist, Scrumptious Fruit Cake
15. Thai-Style Pumpkin, Ginger, Coconut Soup
16. Chocolate Macadamia Roll
17. Rum Balls - without rum
18. Rum Balls - the real thing
19. Apricot Balls
20. Coconut Treats
21. Apricot Fudge
22. High-Energy Treats
23. Pancakes /Strawberry or Blueberry Sauce
24. Strawberry Ginger Cheesecake
25. Kahlua Cheesecake
26. Marshmallow Coconut Fruit
27. Frozen Sinful Stuff
28. Joanna's Cheese Scones
29. Joanna's Tasty Muffins

1. JOANNA'S CHICKEN CASSEROLE

This recipe has been handed from friend to friend so many times that we have no idea where it originated. Joanna, as usual, has made her own improvements.

Ingredients:

1.5kg (3lb) chicken pieces (for best flavor, leave the skin on)

2 cups gluten-free tomato sauce (ketchup)

4 teaspoons oil

2 teaspoons brown sugar

2 large onions OR dried onion

2 teaspoons gluten-free dry mustard

4 cloves garlic OR garlic powder

2 teaspoons gluten-free curry powder

2 teaspoons oil, extra

4 teaspoons gluten-free vinegar

4 teaspoons lemon juice

2 teaspoons gluten-free soy sauce (from health food store)

2 teaspoons grated lemon rind

Salt and freshly ground pepper

Method:

Sauté chicken in hot oil until golden brown, remove from pan, drain. Pour off oil from pan, add all other ingredients. Stir until pan brownings are dissolved. Add chicken. Cook on low heat until tender.

Nice served with rice and green vegetables.

Note: You should have plenty of leftovers for second helpings or to heat up for another day. Freezes well.

2. CHEESE SAUCE (with butter)

Ingredients:

60g (2 oz.) butter

1 tablespoon parmesan

3 level tablespoons maize cornflour (in U.S., cornstarch)

60g (2 oz.) tasty cheese, grated

500ml (2 cups) skim milk

Method:

Melt butter in a pot. Add cornstarch, stir well. Add skim milk. Stir constantly until thickened. Add cheeses. Stir until cheese has melted.

3. SAVOURY RICE BAKE

This is one of those marvelous recipes in which the exact ingredients and proportions don't matter. You can easily adapt it to suit the ingredients you have. If you're making meringues -- or any other recipe using egg whites -- you can throw the extra yolks in the savoury bake.

Ingredients:

5 cups cooked rice

2 tablespoons sharp parmesan

4 eggs, beaten

6 rashers bacon, chopped

500g (1 lb) cottage cheese

250g (8 oz) frozen corn kernels

250g (8 oz) mushrooms chopped

3 medium tomatoes, sliced

2 large chopped onions

1/4 teaspoon salt

4 or 5 medium size tomatoes, chopped freshly ground black pepper

2 cups tasty grated cheese (we use low fat cheese)

Method:

Mix everything (except for 1 cup of the grated cheese and the sliced tomatoes) well. Turn into a greased oven-proof dish. We use one 36x26cm (14x10 inches). Using a smaller, deeper dish is fine -- it will just take longer to cook. Cover the top with slices of tomato and then 1 cup of grated tasty cheese.

Bake at 220 C (400 F) for about 50 minutes until firm and cooked through. Serve with green vegetables or salad. Serves 8 to 10.

Note: You can have lots of fun with this recipe. If you like, leave out the mushrooms and experiment with other vegetables.

We deliberately make far more than we can eat in one meal. The leftovers are excellent for snacks and quick, easy lunches, within a day or two. If frozen, it goes soggy but still tastes great.

4. SALMON AND RICE SOUFFLE

A bit heavier than the usual soufflé, this one won't collapse while you're waiting for people to come and get it.

Ingredients:

425g (about 13oz) tin salmon, drained

1 onion

4 eggs

1 tablespoon butter

2 cups cooked rice

1 teaspoon lemon juice

1 cup milk

salt and pepper

Method:

Melt the butter. Chop up the onion. Mix the salmon, cooked rice, milk, onion, lemon juice and butter. Add salt and pepper to taste.

Separate the eggs. Beat the yolks and add them. Beat the egg whites till stiff and fold them in. Put mixture in a greased oven-proof dish and bake at 190 C (365 F) until it's firm -- about half an hour.

5. CHEESY POTATO AND HAM CASSEROLE

Ingredients:

3 medium potatoes, peeled and thinly sliced.

1/2 cup milk

1 onion sliced

2 tablespoons gluten-free chutney

2 hard-boiled eggs, chopped

1/4 teaspoon paprika

3/4 cup grated tasty cheese

freshly ground black pepper

1/4 cup cooked ham, chopped

herb salt

Method:

Grease an oven-proof dish with half the potato and onion slices. Sprinkle with salt and pepper. Spread the cheese, ham, chutney and eggs over the potato slices. Pour the milk over it. Use the remaining potato and onion slices to make another layer. Add the milk and sprinkle with paprika.

Bake in 180 C (360 f) oven for about 30 minutes. By then, the potatoes should be tender.

Microwave version: Microwave for 15 to 20 minutes.

6. PORK WITH CHERRY ALMOND SAUCE

Yum. We love this. It's a great special treat to serve guests. Make enough to give them second helpings.

Ingredients:

8 pork chops	gluten-free rice syrup
1/4 teaspoon salt	1/4 teaspoon ground cloves
345g (11oz) glace cherries	1/4 cup slivered almonds
1/4 teaspoon nutmeg	1/4 teaspoon cinnamon
1/4 cup golden syrup OR	1/4 cup red wine vinegar
	1/8 teaspoon black pepper

Method:

While the pork chops are frying, combine the cherries, golden syrup, vinegar, salt, pepper and spices. Bring to boil and boil for one minute. Add the almonds and pour a third of the sauce over the frying chops. Pour the remaining sauce over the chops when serving.

Serve with fresh steamed vegetables.

7. ASPARAGUS IN CRAB SAUCE

Ingredients:

155g (5oz) gluten-free rice vermicelli	4 bunches of fresh asparagus
2 cups chicken stock, homemade OR made	2 tablespoons maize cornstarch
220g (7oz) canned crab meat with gluten-free stock cubes	2 teaspoons peanut oil

Method:

Boil rice vermicelli for about 10 minutes. Heat oil in a pan and add chopped asparagus. Stir-fry for 5 minutes. Add chicken stock and cornstarch, add crab meat. Stir until sauce is thick. Pour over vermicelli and serve.

8. FAST BEEF STROGANOFF (microwave)

So easy - so tasty.

Ingredients:

500kg (1/2 pound) ground beef

3 1/2 cups hot water

1 packet gluten-free onion soup mix

1 can sliced mushrooms

3 cups gluten-free rice noodles

1 cup cream

1/2 teaspoons ground ginger cornstarch

Method:

Microwave ground beef on HIGH for 5 minutes. Add packet of soup, noodles, ginger, hot water. Cook 12 minutes. Add mushrooms and cream and thicken with cornstarch. Microwave for another minute.

9. BACON, POTATO AND ONION PIE

Ingredients:

2 large potatoes, thinly slice

2 eggs

2 large onions, sliced

pepper and herb salt

6 rashers of bacon

1 cup milk

Method:

Place layers in a greased oven-proof dish in this order: onion, bacon, potato. Repeat. Top layer should be potato.

Beat two eggs, add seasoning. Add milk and pour over the layers. Bake in oven at 190C (375F) until the top browns.

10. SALMON AND POTATO BAKE

Ingredients:

440g (14oz) tinned salmon

1/2 cup cream

500g (1 point) potatoes, boiled and sliced

1 small onion, finely chopped

60g (2oz) butter

1 teaspoon gluten-free dry mustard

3 tablespoons flour

1/2 cup tasty cheese, grated

1 1/2 cups milk

1/2 cup gluten-free cornflakes

3 tablespoons cornstarch

1/2 teaspoon paprika

Method:

Melt the butter in a saucepan, add the flour and cook for one minute. Add the cream and milk and gently bring to a boil, stirring constantly until the sauce thickens.

Remove from stove and add the mustard, half the cheese and gently fold in the salmon. Avoid mashing it.

In an oven-proof dish, arrange alternative layers of potato slices and the salmon mixture. Sprinkle cornflakes over the top, followed by the remaining cheese and paprika.

Bake in 180 C (360 F) oven for about half an hour until nicely golden brown on top. Serve with green vegetables or salad.

11. TROPICAL CHICKEN

Ingredients:

1 tablespoon olive oil

1 tablespoon gluten-free tomato sauce

500g (1 pound) raw chicken, in small chunks

1/4 cup water

1 medium onion, chopped

1 gluten-free chicken stock cube

1 bell pepper, sliced

1 banana, sliced

1 tablespoon cornstarch

1 or 2 tsp gluten-free curry powder, to suit your taste buds

440g (14oz) unsweetened tinned pineapple, including juice

Method:

In a non-stick frypan, heat the oil and fry the chicken, onion and bell pepper for about four minutes. Stir so it doesn't burn.

Blend the cornstarch and curry powder in a little of the water, add tomato sauce and remaining water. Add to the frypan with stock cube, canned pineapple and pineapple juice.

Stir until the sauce boils and thickens. Lower the heat, cover and simmer for 20 minutes. Just before serving add sliced banana. Serve with rice.

12. RICE TOMATO PILAF

Every keen cook seems to have his or her own ideas on how rice should be cooked. Some say it must be washed first, some say it should never be washed or rinsed after cooking, and some suggest soaking it in water for at least two hours before it is cooked. Whichever way you prepare it, here's a way to add lots of flavour.

Ingredients:

30g (1 oz.) butter

1/2 teaspoon freshly ground black pepper

2 cups white rice

1 teaspoon cumin

1/2 cup wild rice

2 bay leaves

1 teaspoon salt

1 teaspoon coriander

3 cups tomato juice

Method:

Bring water to a boil, add rice and wild rice. Add everything else. Simmer gently until all the water is absorbed -- about 15 minutes. Cover and let it stand a few minutes.

Serve with salad and cold meat.

13. EASY SALMON FRITATA

The exact ingredients and proportions don't matter too much in this recipe, which is easily adapted to suit your taste buds - and the ingredients you have. You can throw in tinned corn instead of frozen, tuna instead of salmon, and shallots instead of the onion. If you don't have fresh mint or basil, you can use a tablespoon of dried basil.

Ingredients:

4 eggs

1 bell pepper chopped

185g (6oz) can salmon

several sprigs fresh mint or basil chopped

440g (14oz) frozen corn kernels

freshly ground black pepper

1 onion, halved and then sliced

herb salt OR ordinary salt

2 large tomatoes, chopped

1 teaspoon olive oil

Method:

In a heavy frypan, heat the olive oil and cook the chopped onion till it softens. Add the corn, salmon (drained), chopped tomatoes and chopped bell pepper. Stir to combine but don't be too vigorous, you don't want the salmon mashed - try to keep it in small pieces. Sprinkle with pepper, herb salt and chopped mint.

Beat the eggs lightly and pour over the mixture. Cook at very low heat until the eggs are cooked, which will be about 12 minutes.

Serve with fresh green salad.

14. RICH, MOIST, SCRUMPTIOUS FRUIT CAKE (easy to make in a microwave)

I first tasted one of Joanna's delicious fruit cakes about 20 years ago, before we were married. It was beautifully moist, and crammed with lovely fruit and nuts. How could I resist a girl who could bake like that?

After we married, I discovered that her idea of a perfect holiday involves the following essential ingredients: just the two of us, a peaceful, quiet spot, preferably with a view of water, as little physical exercise as possible, a carton of books and a generous supply of food - always including an enormous fruit cake. I must admit I adapted very quickly to the idea.

Over the years, her recipe for a successful holiday has stayed the same, but she has kept experimenting with, and improving, the fruit cake recipe. Not only does it now have several new ingredients, but it can be made quickly and easily in a microwave. A few years ago, she adapted it again, making it gluten-free.

Ingredients:

1kg mixed fruit

1 teaspoons cream of tartar

125g (4oz) butter

1 teaspoon bicarbonate of soda

4 eggs beaten

1 cup bought gluten-free flour OR

1 dessert spoon Parisian essence (brown coloring, optional)

1/2 soya, 1/4 rice and 1/4 potato flour

1 tablespoon nutmeg

440g (14oz) unsweetened crushed Pineapple

1 tablespoon mixed spice

1 tablespoon Amaretto liqueur

125g (4oz) almonds

1 tablespoon Cointreau

1 teaspoon pre-gel starch OR xanthan gum OR guar gum (If you don't have these liqueurs on hand you can buy a nip of each from your local pub, OR whatever liqueurs you prefer OR use almond essence and orange essence)

Method:

Cook the fruit and liqueurs on HIGH for five minutes in the microwave. (Joanna cunningly uses a round glass dish about eight inches wide and four inches deep-20x10cm- and also cooks the cake in it)

Add the butter and spices. Tip this mixture into a large basin and stir in the rest of the ingredients.

Line the glass dish with baking paper, pour in the ingredients, cook on HIGH for 15 minutes, elevating the dish while cooking, for example by sitting it on a small upturned china dish.

Test with a skewer. (When the skewer comes out clean, the cake is cooked)

Allow the cake to cool before removing from the container. You can simply remove the baking paper and put the cake bake in the dish it was cooked in, put the lid on and store in the fridge. How's that for simplicity!

If you can ignore the mouth-watering aroma after a few days the taste improves as the flavors meld together.

15. THAI-STYLE PUMPKIN, GINGER AND COCONUT SOUP

Even if you don't like pumpkin, I think you'll be impressed with this Thai style soup - as long as you like ginger and garlic.

Ingredients:

1 medium size pumpkin	cooking oil
1 large brown onion	stock cubes
1 can coconut cream	herb salt, pepper
3 cloves garlic	2 rounded dessert spoons of ginger in syrup OR fresh ginger
Chicken stock, home-made OR made with gluten-free	

Method:

Remove the pumpkin skin and seeds, chop pumpkin into chunks. Slice onion. Crush garlic. In a large frypan or pan, sauté the onion and garlic in a little oil until golden. Add chunks of pumpkin and sauté, stirring, for five minutes. Add enough chicken stock to cover the pumpkin. Add ginger.

Bring to a boil and then simmer for about 15 minutes, till the pumpkin is soft. Take it off the heat and allow to cool. Blend the mixture to a puree.

Put it back on the stove, add coconut cream and salt and pepper. Bring the heat up slowly until the soup is simmering. Adjust seasoning to taste.

16. CHOCOLATE MACADAMIA ROLL

Ingredients:

250g (8oz) rice cookies
(from health food shop)

60g (2oz) butter

1/2 cup raisins, chopped

1 egg

1/2 cup macadamia nuts,
chopped

2 tbls Amaretto OR liqueur
of your choice

155g (5oz) dark chocolate

Method:

Crush cookies, not too finely. Melt chocolate with
Amaretto. Beat the eggs, and combine with butter,
melted, then combine with chocolate mixture. Mix well.

Work mixture into a sausage shape, place on aluminum
foil and roll up into lengths. Chill until it's firm. Dust with
icing sugar and cut into slices. If there's any left over -
there probably won't be - keep it in the fridge.

Note: the consistency of the mixture may vary depending
on the brand of gluten-free biscuits used. If it seems too
sloppy, try putting in the fridge for a few hours before
rolling into lengths.

17. RUM BALLS - WITHOUT RUM

These are quick and easy to make

Ingredients:

200g (6 1/2oz) gluten-free rice cookies (from health food shop)

60g (2oz) glace cherries, chopped

400g (13oz) condensed skim milk

2 tablespoons cocoa

1 cup dried coconut

1 tablespoon butter rum essence

1/2 cup shredded coconut

1 cup mixed dried fruit extra dried coconut

Method:

Crush rice cookies in food processor. If you don't have one, put cookies in a sturdy plastic bag, tie it up leaving as little air as possible inside, place bag on floor an use your heal to crush cookies.

Mix all ingredients in a large bowl. The consistency may vary depending on the brand of biscuits used. If it seems too sloppy, refrigerate it for a few hours. Roll into small balls - guests tend to look for a small ball to sample, then return for a larger one. Roll balls in dried coconut. Refrigerate. If you can manage to leave them alone, the taste improves when the flavors have melded for a day or two.

Variations: You may like to try them flavored with walnuts and a tablespoon of strong black coffee, or almonds and almond essence.

The original recipe had no cherries, no fruit, less coconut and two tablespoons of rum. I'd love to hear how our experiments turn out.

18. RUM BALLS-THE REAL THING

Bundaberg Rum is produced in Queensland. It's potent stuff. Easy to make, these sweet treats are a nice perk-me-up served with a late-night cup of coffee.

Ingredients:

250g (8oz) dark chocolate

2 tablespoon butter

4 teaspoons overproof rum - from Bundagerg, of course!

2 tablespoon sweetened condensed skim milk

2 teaspoon vanilla essence cocoa

Method:

Melt chocolate and butter over hot water. Stir in condensed milk. Beat in rum and vanilla. Chill until firm enough to handle. Using a teaspoon, form balls and drop into cocoa. Store in refrigerator.

19. APRICOT BALLS

Ingredients:

Rind from 1/2 orange

1/4 cup fresh orange juice

1/2 cup super fine sugar

11/2 cups dried coconut

250g (8oz) dried apricots, chopped finely

extra coconut

Method:

Grate the rind, add sugar, dried apricot, juice and coconut. Blend. You need enough coconut to make frim balls which hold together. Form into small balls. You'll need to wet your fingers frequently to stop the balls from sticking.

Roll balls in extra coconut. Refrigerate

Variation: Replace some of the orange juice with apricot brandy.

20. COCONUT TREATS

These have become a favorite snack in our home - great with a cup of coffee.

Ingredients:

2 cups shredded coconut

125g (4oz) gluten-free chocolate chips

2 cups dried coconut

100g (6 1/2 oz.) chopped dried apricots

1 tin sweetened condensed skim milk

Method:

Mix coconut and condensed milk. Divide mixture in half. Add chocolate chips to one half of mixture, and add dried apricots to the other half. Mix well.

Dollop teaspoonfuls of mixture on to a non-stick baking tray. Bake at 150 C (325 F) until slightly golden.

Variety: Dried mango works well instead of dried apricots.

Note: You may have to experiment with the cooking time: you can have them golden and crisp or only slightly golden and still chewy. Yum!

21. APRICOT FUDGE

Ingredients:

185g (6oz) brown sugar

2 cups dried apricots, chopped

250g (8oz) butter

2 packets gluten-free rice cookies, crushed

400g (13oz) condensed skim milk

Method:

Slowly heat the sugar, butter and condensed milk until it's smooth and well blended. Add the dried apricots and crushed biscuits. Mix well and spread in a sponge roll tin.

Refrigerate.

22. HIGH-ENERGY TREATS

Ingredients:

1 cup almonds

1 tablespoon honey OR gluten-free rice syrup

1 cup mixed dried apricots

and dates

sesame seeds

Juice of 1 orange

Method:

Chop the nuts and dried fruit thoroughly, by hand or in a food processor. Add the honey and fruit juice. (If it's a large juicy orange, don't use all the juice - drink some.) Roll into balls the size of walnuts. Roll in sesame seeds (may be lightly toasted first.) Refrigerate.

Variations: Add a dash of your favorite liqueur. Use your choice of other dried fruit.

23. PANCAKES WITH BLUEBERRY OR STRAWBERRY SAUCE

Pancake ingredients:

1 cup brown rice flour

1 cup white rice flour

1 1/4 cups water

2 eggs

Pancake method:

Blend everything except the eggs in a food processor. Allow the mixture to stand for at least two hours.

Add the eggs and beat. Brush a frying pan with oil. Pour in some of the mixture. Cover with a lid and cook on medium low heat about five minutes. Turn with a spatula and cook the other side.

Strawberry filling ingredients:

300ml (1/2 pint) cream

500g (1 pound) strawberries (may substitute blueberries)

1/4 cup lemon juice

100g (1/4 tin) condensed skim milk

Method:

Spread the filling thickly on the pancakes, roll up, and serve. Put a dollop more on top.

24. STRAWBERRY GINGER CHEESECAKE

Base ingredients:

1 packet gluten-free rice cookies OR gluten-free Cornflakes

90g (3oz) butter

1 teaspoon cinnamon

1 teaspoon ground ginger

Base method:

Blend all ingredients in a food processor. Press into a dish and place in fridge while you make the strawberry topping.

Strawberry topping ingredients:

300 (1/2 pint) cream

1/4 cup lemon juice

100g (1/4 tin) unsweetened condensed skim milk

500g (1pound) strawberries

Method:

Add the topping to the base and refrigerate.

25. KAHLUA CHEESECAKE

You can make this delicious cheesecake with just a hint of liqueur or lots, depending on individual taste.

Ingredients:

Base:

125g (4oz) gluten-free rice cookies OR gluten-free cornflakes, crushed

45g (1 1/2 oz.) butter, melted

Filling:

2 teaspoons gelatin

2 tablespoons superfine sugar

1 1/2 tablespoons hot water

200g (1/2 tin) sweetened condensed skim milk

125ml (4oz.) cream, whipped

60 to 85ml (2 to 2 1/2 oz.) Kahlua

375g (12oz) cream cheese

Topping:

60g (2oz) dark chocolate, melted

Method:

Mix the crushed rice cookies and melted butter and press on to the base and sides of small dish

Refrigerate.

Dissolve the gelatin in hot water. Whip the cream and put aside. Blend the cream cheese and sugar until smooth. Add the condensed milk and liqueur and fold in the cream and gelatin.

Melt the chocolate in microwave, stir, and swirl into the mixture. Pour mixture on to the crust and refrigerate overnight.

Serve with cream or ice cream

26. MARSHMALLOW COCONUT FRUIT

You can eat this either as a dessert or with a salad. If you're making it for a crowd, make plenty.

People will come back for more. Warning: make sure that the marshmallows you use are Gluten-free. They often aren't. You can use fresh or canned pineapple and mandarin pieces.

Ingredients:

440g (14oz) pineapple pieces, drained

1 cup seedless grapes

220g (7oz) mandarin pieces

2 cups sour cream

220g (7oz) gluten-free marshmallows teaspoon salt

125g (4 oz) dried or flaked coconut

Method:

Combine everything in a bowl and chill overnight.

Alternative suggested by Deanna Polakowski (DeannaP@ cris.com) "Add 1 large bottle of drained maraschino cherries. Besides adding another flavor to the recipe, they also make it a very festive pink color."

27. FROZEN SINFUL STUFF

Who could say no to this memorable dessert? It's delightfully rich and creamy, fruity and spicy. Joanna thinks it's too creamy.

Ingredients:

600ml (1 pint) whipping cream

90b (3oz) glace cherries, halved

1 cup mixed dried fruit

60g (2oz) flaked almonds, lightly toasted

200g (7oz) condensed skim milk

1/4 cup Amaretto liqueur OR brandy

155g (5oz) dark cooking chocolate

3/4 teaspoon mixed spice

Method:

Soak mixed dried fruit in liqueur for at least an hour - preferably overnight.

Break chocolate into small pieces and melt in microwave on HIGH for 1 minute 45 seconds, or in heat- proof bowl over simmering water.

Whip the cream - not too much, you don't want to make butter. Stir in condensed milk and melted chocolate. Add mixed fruit, glace cherries, nuts and mixed spice. Stir thoroughly. Freeze in a two-liter container.

Now for the hardest part: be patient. You'll need to wait at least eight hours before it's ready to enjoy.

28. JOANNA'S CHEESE SCONES

My wife Joanna is the expert on the scones in our house. She produces some delightfully tasty ones with this recipe which she created.

Ingredients:

1 egg

2 cups grated, tasty, low-fat cheese

3 cups gluten-free (commercial mix) flour

1 tablespoon grated parmesan

5 teaspoons gluten-free baking powder

pinch cayenne

Method:

Beat the egg with 3/4 to 1 cup of milk. Mix remaining ingredients with as little handling as possible.

Bake at 450 F (230 C)+ for 10 minutes.

29. JOANNA'S TASTY MUFFINS

(English? Well, not exactly)

As above, add chopped bacon, corn, extra egg and extra milk (half to three-quarters of a cup). Yes, I know that's all awfully imprecise, but that's the way Joanna is when it comes to cooking. Good Luck.

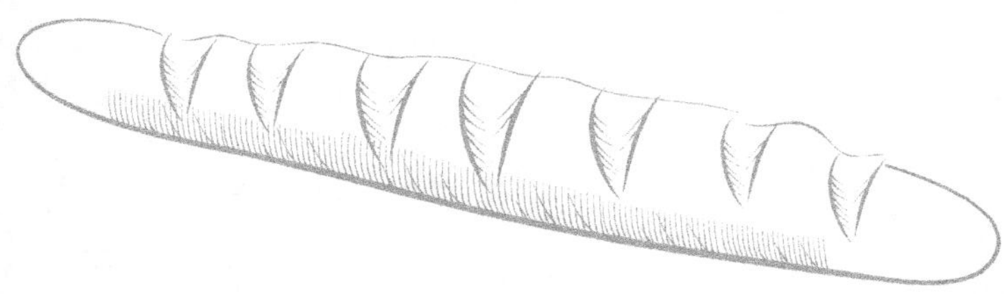

TO ORDER GLUTEN FREE PRODUCTS

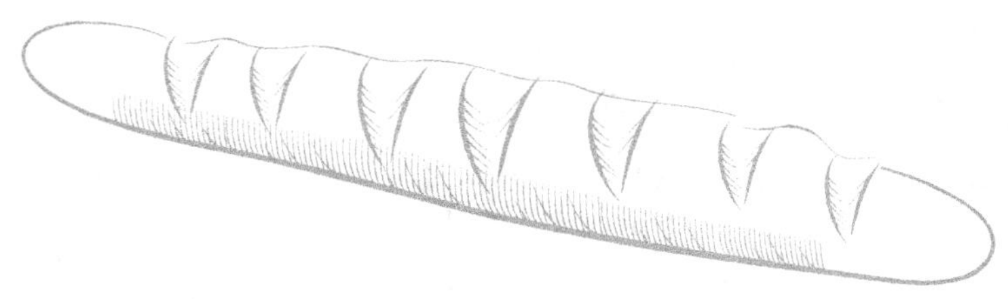

TO ORDER GLUTEN FREE PRODUCTS

Bickford Flavors, 19007 St. Clair Ave., Cleveland, OH 44117, (216) 531-6006

Blue Diamond Growers, 4800 Sisk Rd., Modesto, CA., 95356., (209) 545-6229, Fax (209) 545-6215

Bob Red Mill Natural Foods, 5209 S.E. International Way, Milwaukie, OR 97222 (503) 645-3215

CEMAC Foods, 1281 E. Sedgley Ave., Philadelphia, PA 19124, (800) 724-0179, (215) 288-7440

Carolina Country Kitchen, Inc., P.O. Box 1371, Flat Rock, NC 28731-1371 (828) 693-6549, E-Mail: cck@brinet.com, Web: www. brinet.com/~cck

Chef Evan, Web: www.chefevan.com

Conrad Rice Mill, Inc., 307 Ann St., New Iberia, LA 70562 (800) 551-3245

Cybros, Inc., PO Box 851, Waukesha, WI 53187, (800) 876-2253

Darla M. Gennings, 6026 Blue Mist Lane, Dallas, TX 75248, (214) 733-0172

DeBoles Nutritional Foods, Inc., 215 Hillside Ave., Williston Park, NY, (516) 742-1252

Dietary Specialties, PO Box 227, Rochester, NY 14601, (800) 544-0099 Web: www.dietspec.com

Ener-G Foods, Inc., PO Box 84487, Seattle WA 98124-5787, (800) 331-5222 Web: www.ener-g.com

Floyds of Denver, Box 636, Littleton, Colorado 80160 (303) 730-7197 E-Mail: floydsofdenv@earthlink.net

Foods By George, 530 Broad Street, Glen Rock, NJ 07452, (201) 612-9700

Food-For-Life Baking Co., 2991 E. Doherty St., Corona, CA 91719 (800) 797-5090, Web: www.food-for.life.com

Freeda Vitamins, Inc., 3 East 41st St., New York, New NY 10017 (800) 777-3737, (212) 685-4980, E-Mail: Freedavits@aol.com

Frookie, 2070 Maple St., Des Plaines, IL 60018 (888) 376-0543 Web: www.frookie.com

F.T. Loa Cookies, 551 Valley Rd., Suite 124, Upper Montclair, NJ 07043 (888) 366-8709, Fax: (888) 366-8709, Web: www. ftloacookies.com

G! Foods, 3536 17th St., San Francisco, CA 94110, (415) 255-2139 Web: www.g-foods.com

Garden Spot Distributors, 438 White Oaks, New Holland, PA 17557, (800) 829-5100

G&I Kosher Bakery, 130-10 180th St., Springfield Gardens, NY 11434, (718) 481-7000, Fax: (718) 481-8811

Gillian's Foods, 462 Proctor Ave., Revere MA. 02151-5730, (718) 286-4095, E-Mail: R357BOBO@aol.com Web: www.Gillians-Foods.com

The Gluten-Free Cookie Jar, PO Box 52, Trevose, PA 19053, (215) 355-9403

Gluten Free Delights, P.O. Box, 284, Cedar Falls, Iowa, 50613, (319) 266-7167 Web: www.quikpage.com/G/glutenfree

The Gluten-Free Pantry, PO Box 840, Glastonburry, CT 06033, (203) 633-3826 (800) 291-8386, E-Mail: orders@glurtenfree. com, Web: www.glutenfree.com

David Goodbatters', P.O. Box 102 Dept. M, Bausman, PA 17504, (717) 872-0652

Heartymix, 1231 Madison Hill Rd., Rahway, NJ 07065, (908) 382-0652

Jowar Foods, 5608 83rd, Lubbock, TX 79424, (806) 363-9070 E-Mail: rlmiler@cy-net.com Web: www.jowar.com

Just Devine GF Cakes & Sweets, 4820 Tabard Pl, Annadale, VA 22003 (703) 425-7899

King Arthur Flour, RR 2, Box 56, Norwich, VT 05055, (800) 827-6836

Lang Naturals, 741 Namquid Drive, Warwick, RI, 02888, (800) 728-2348
Web: freeleaf.ne.mediaone.net/LANGweb/gifttin.html

Little Market Moon, 715 SE 46th, Portland, OR 97215, (503) 232-8980

Mendocino Gluten-Free Products, Inc., Willits, CA, (800) 297-5399 E-Mail: jbwade@innovation.com Web: www.zapcom. net/~jbwade

MenuDirect, 865 Centennial, Piscataway, NJ 08854, (888) 636-8123 Web: www.menudirect.com

Mrs. Leeper's Pasta, 12455 Kerran St, #200, Poway, CA 92064 (760) 486-1101

Miss Roben's, PO Box 1434, Frederick, MD 21702, (800) 891-0083 Web: www.jagunet.com/~msrobens E-Mail: missroben@ aol.com

Natural Feast Corp, PO Box 50158 New Bedford MA 02745, (508) 984-4230

Natural Highlights, PO Box 3526, Chico, CA 95927, (800) 313-6454

Omega Nutrition, 1720 Labountry Rd., Ferndale, WA 98248, (800) 661-3529 E-Mail: Omega@istar.ca

Old Windmill Specialty Foods, 5014 16th Ave., Suite 202, Brooklyn, NY 11204 (800) 653-3791

OroWest Foods, PO Box 50301, Eugene, OR 97405, (541) 484-1010

Pamela Products, 156 Utah Avenue So., So. San Francisco, CA 94080, (415) 952-4546

Patti Pastries, 1211 Tree St., Philadelphia, PA 19148, (215) 336-5004

Prote-Grab, 6045 NW 82nd Dr, Miami, FL., (305) 392-5035 Fax: (305) 392-5038, Web: www.protegrab.com.ar/kapac
The Really Great Food Company, PO Box 319, Malberne, NY 11565, (800) 593-5377 (516) 593-5587

Red Mill Farms, 290 South 5th Street, Brooklyn, NY 11211, (718) 384-2150

S&B Gezunt, Inc., 585 Harwood Ave, Satellite Beach, FL 32937 E-Mail: bchefer@sprynet.com Web: home.sprynet.com/sprynet/bchefer

Schiffy III Catering, 19 Hanover Pl., Ste 313, Hicksville, NY 11801-5103, (516) 681-0895

Shilo Farms, PO Bo 97, Solphur Springs, AK 72768, (501) 298-3297

Solgar Vitamin & Herb Co., 500 Willow Tree Rd., Leonia, NJ 070605 (201) 944-2312, Web: www.solgar.com/online_reference/food_sens/index.html

Sterk's Bakery, 1402 Pine Ave. STE 542, Niagara Falls, NY 14301, (800) 608-4501

Stokes Medical Arts Pharmacy, 639 Stokes Rd., Medford, NJ 08055 (800) 745-5222 Web: www.stokesrx.com E-Mail: stokes-rx@cyberenet.net

Tad Enterprises, 9356 Pleasant, Tinley Park, IL 60477 (708) 429-2101

Tamarind Tree, Ltd., 1037 State Street, Perth Amboy, NJ 08871, (800) 432-8733 Fax: (908) 293-1507, Web: www.tamtree.com E-Mail: tamtree@bellatlantic.net

Ultimate Biscotti, 1000 S. Bertelsen Rd. #10, Eugene, OR 97402, E-Mail: info@ultimatebiscotti.com Web: www.ultimatebiscotti.com

Vans International, 20318 Gramercy Pl., Torrance, CA 90501, (310) 320-8611

Walnut Acres, Penns Creek: PA 17862, (800) 433-3998 Web: www.walnutacres.com

Watkins, service by local distributors: (Kent Rogers, 13028 Powell Rd, Wake Forest, NC 27587; (888) 556-7235, E-Mail: RogersGrp@aol.com)

Whyte's Darifree (Garden-Good Things Ltd.) E-mail: Darifree@darifree.com Web: www.darifree.com

Canada

Nelson David of Canada, 101-193 Dumolin ST., Winnipeg, Manitoba R2H 0E4 (204) 237-9161

De-Ro-Ma (1983) Lte, 910, Boul, Jarry Daval, Que, Canada H7W 2W6, (514) 687-2287, (800) 236-3438, Fax: (514) 687-2289, E-Mail: deroma@odyssee.net Web: www.cosmo2000.ca/deroma

El Peto Products, 2-41 Shoemaker St., Kitchener, Ontario N2E 3G9 (800) 387-4064, (519) 748-5211, E-Mail: elpeto@golden.net

Food Directions Inc., 15 Milner Ave, Units 121-23, Scarborough, Ontario, Canada M1S 3R3, Web: www.tinkyada.com

Grain Process Enterprises, 39 Golden Gate Ct., Scarborough, Ontario M1P 3A4 (416) 291-3226

Kaybee Gluten-Free Products, Box 829, Cudworth, Saskatchewan S0K 1B0 Phone/Fax: (306) 256-3424

Kinnikinnik Foods, 10306-112 Street, Edmonton, AB, CA T5K 1N1 (403) 424-2900, Fax: (403) 421-0456, Orders: (877) 503-4466 E-Mail: info@kinnikinnick.com Web: www.sas.ab.ca/kinnikinnick

Kingsmill Foods Company Limited, 1399 Kenedy Road, Unit #17, Scarborough, Ontario Canada, M1P 2L6 (416) 755-1124

Liv-N-Well Distributors Ltd., #1-7900 River Road, Richmond B.C. V6X 1X7 Canada (604) 270-8474, Fax: (604) 270-1147, E-Mail: zeno@direct.ca

Natural Products INC., 143 Elman Cres., New Market, Ontario, L3Y 7X2

Nature's Path Foods, Inc. 7453 Progress Way, Delta, BC VG 1E8, E-Mail: Cereal@naturespath.bc.ca

Nelson David of Canada, 101-193 Dumolin St., Winnipeg, Manitoba R2H 0E4 (204) 237-9161

Panne Rizo Rice Breads, 1939 Cornwall Ave, Vancouver, BC
V6J 1C8 (604) 736-0885, Fax: (604) 736-0825, E-Mail: sallay@
PanneRizoRiceBreads.com

Pastariso Products, 55 Ironside Crescent, Units 6&7, Scarborough Ontario M1X 1N3 (416) 321-9090

Rice Innovations Inc., Pickering Postal Station, PO Box 16, Pickering, Ontario Canada L1V 2R2

Son's Milling, Unit #11, 130 Dallas Rd., Victoria BCV V8V 1A3
(604) 389-6743

Specialty Foods, Hospital for Sick Children, 555 University Ave
Toronto, Onmt, (800-737-7976), (416) 813-1500
875 Main St.W., Hamilton, (905) 528-4707

Sterk's Bakery, 3866 23rd St., Vineland, Ontario L0R 2C0,
(905) 562-3086

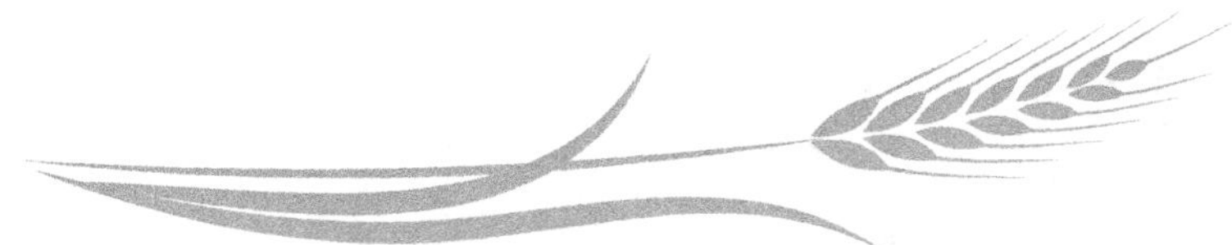

CELIAC DISEASE RESOURCES

National Foundation for Celiac Awareness
124 South Maple Street
Ambler, PA 19002
Phone: (215) 325-1306
Email: Info@celiaccentral.org
Internet: www.celiaccentral.org

North American Society for Pediatric Gastroenterology, Hepatology and Nutrition (NASPGHAN)
P.O. Box 6
Flourtown, PA 19031
Phone: (215) 233-0808
Fax: (215) 233-3918
Email: naspghan@naspghan.org
Internet: www.naspghan.org ; www.cdhnf.org

National Digestive Diseases Information Clearinghouse (NDDIC)
2 Information Way
Bethesda, MD 20892-3570
Phone: 1-800-891-5389
Fax: (703) 738-4929
Email: nddic@info.niddk.nih.gov
Internet: www.digestive.niddk.nih.gov

America Celiac Society
59 Crystal Ave
West Orange, NJ 07052-4114
Phone: (973) 325-8837
Email: americeliacsoc@netscape.net

Celiac Sprue Association USA
PO Box 31700
Omaha, NE 68131-0700
Phone: (412) 558-0600
Email: celiacs@csaceliacs.org
Internet: www.csaceliacs.org

Gluten Intolerance Group
15110 10th Ave. SW, Suite A
Seattle, WA 98166-1820
Phone: (206) 246-6652
Email: info@gluten.net; gig@gluten.net

Celiac Disease Foundation
13251 Ventura Blvd. Suite 1
Studio City, CA 91604-1838
Phone: (818) 990-2354
Email: cdf@celiac.org
Internet: www.celiac.org

Gluten Free Living
P.O. Box 105
Hastings-on-Hudson, NY 10706
Email: gfliving@aol.com

Canadian Celiac Association
190 Britannia Rd. East, Unit 11
Mississauga, Ontario, Canada L4Z 1W6
Phone: (905) 507-6208 | (800) 363-7296
Internet: www.celiac.ca

The Food Allergy Network
10400 Eaton Place, Suite 107
Fairfax, VA 22030-2208
Phone: 1-800-929-4040
Email: faan@foodallergy.org
Internet: Foodallergy.org

American Dietetic Association
216 W. Jackson Blvd.
Chicago, IL 60606-6995
Phone: (312) 899-0040 | (800) 366-1655
Email: hotline@eatright.org
Internet: www.eatright.org

Living Without
PO Box 2126
Northbrook, IL 60065
Phone: (847) 480-8810
Internet: www.livingwithout.com

REFERENCES

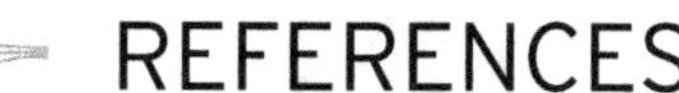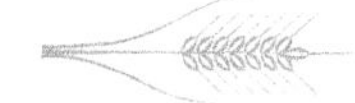

Communique - A Mayo Reference Services Publication, Volume 26 No.12 December 2001.

The National Digestive Diseases Information Clearing House (NDDIC) - A service of the National Institute of Diabetes and Digestive and Kidney Diseases.

Established in 1980, the Clearing House provides information about digestive diseases to people with digestive disorders and to their families, health care professionals and the public.

If you wish to perform your own search of the database, you may access and search the NDDIC Reference Collection Database online.

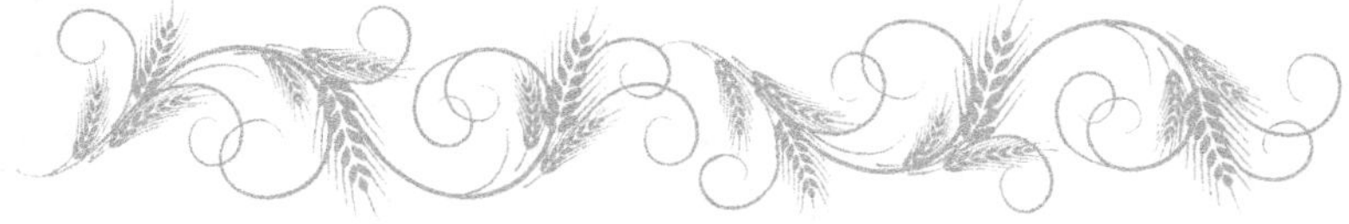